Color Me Healthy

By **William Campbell Douglass II**, MD

Rhino Publishing, S.A.

Color Me Healthy

ISBN 9962-636-10-8

Cover illustration by
María Luisa Gutiérrez
and
Alex Manyoma (alex@3dcity.com)

Please, visit Rhino's website for other publications from
Dr. William Campbell Douglass
www.rhinopublish.com

Dr. Douglass' "Real Health" alternative medical newsletter is available at www.realhealthnews.com

RHINO PUBLISHING, S.A.
World Trade Center
Panama, Republic of Panama
Voicemail/Fax
International: + 416-352-5126
North America: 888-317-6767

Table of Contents

Introduction

"In neglected light and color, there is a potency far beyond that of drugs and serums."
— Kate W. Baldwin, M.D., 1927

"He's crazy!"

"He's got to be a quack!"

"Who gave this guy his medical license?"

"He's a nut case!"

In case you're wondering, those are the reactions you'll probably get if you show your doctor this report. I know the idea of healing many common ailments simply by exposing them to colored light sounds far-fetched, but when you see the evidence, you'll agree that color is truly an amazing medical breakthrough.

When I first heard the stories, I reacted much the same way. But the evidence so convinced me, that I had to try color therapy in my practice. My results were truly amazing. Here's just one example: A Croatian woman, brought in by her son, who acted as interpreter, had an ulcer the size of a silver dollar on the side of her leg, just below the knee. It was a half-inch deep and full of pus.

She recounted to me five long, terrible years of unsuccessful treatments for the open ulcer on her leg. She had tried everything: salves, unguents, potions, and antibiotics. But nothing worked.

Doctors had even treated it with surgery (debridement, i.e., scraping) for *one year* with no discernible result. By the time she came to see me, the family was desperate and willing to try anything. They had heard that I used some strange light therapies and wanted to give me a chance.

We treated the ulcer with Indigo color and, after being sure her son understood the technique, we had him treat her at home for an hour, twice a day. Within days, new skin growth had begun to cover the open sore and she was free from pain within a week. They came to see me six weeks later with the ulcer almost completely healed!

I know it's hard to believe, but color therapy really works. And not just for external wounds. It also works for many internal ailments at which modern medicine just throws useless drugs and surgery. If you're still having trouble believing me, sit back and listen to the following story.

Chapter 1

Where It All Began

Dinshah Ghadiali, a young Indian physician fresh out of training, was awakened in the middle of the night by a loud pounding on his door. A young barefoot boy had been sent by his mistress, a prominent lady of the city, to fetch him. The boy, wide-eyed and breathless, said his mistress was surely dying and Dinshah must come at once. He dressed, got on his bicycle and dashed through the heavy tropical night.

The woman had severe "colitis," probably cholera, and could hardly speak. "Dinshah" she whispered, "please save me; I am about to die." She had been to the best professors of the city, as befitted a woman of her station, even though she knew of Dinshah's reputation as a remarkable young healer. A number of toxic medications, including mercury (this was 1897) sat on the bedside table. She was having 50 bowel movements a day, undoubtedly made worse by the nostrums provided by Dinshah's learned professional betters. It was clear that she would die if something dramatic and unorthodox wasn't done, and done soon, he thought.

In this dimly lit room, with a prominent patient dying before him, Dinshah was seized with a sense of panic and helplessness. If he gathered the courage to do what he knew needed to be done — take her off the killing drugs and try a different, unorthodox approach — *he* would be blamed for her death. Dinshah had an unfortunate combination of qualities for any doctor who wants to practice medicine and "get along," but, at the same time, do what he thinks is right for his patients: he was stubborn, honorable and courageous. He did what he felt had to be done.

As the wide-eyed servant boy watched, Dinshah swept all the medicine bottles into the bedside wastebasket. He ordered his patient to take nothing but water and dashed for the door, saying he would be back with a remedy to cure her, knowing in his heart and saying to himself: "I am a miserable charlatan — only divine intervention can save this woman."

Dinshah walked briskly through the dark early morning air. There was a dim promise of sunlight causing ghostly silhouettes on the trees to the East. He ploughed through his memories, his list of ancient Indian lore and his medical catechism. He prayed to his Indian gods, seeking a direction. The name of Dr. Edwin D. Babbitt dropped into his mind. "Color!" he thought. The healing power of color!

Dr. Babbitt had written a treatise on the use of colors, externally applied, in the treatment of disease in 1876. The work, entitled *The Principles of Light and Color*, had always held a fascination for Dinshah. It had been tucked away in the recesses of his mind for future consideration. The future was now — and it would change the course of his life. He would never turn back.

There was a road construction ahead and the workers had not yet arrived to turn off the Indigo-colored glass lanterns used to warn passing carriages and horsemen of the hazard of road excavations and equipment. Dinshah looked around furtively like a common thief, grabbed the nearest lantern, extinguished the light, and ran at full speed back to the mansion and his dying patient.

The young doctor, with sweat running from his face and breathing intensely, turned the lamp on at it's highest intensity to get the maximum of the deep Violet-Blue light to bathe the bare abdomen of his barely breathing patient. He rubbed her limbs, talked softly to her and, with a feeling of shame, told her that the worst would soon be over and she would be well again.

With the application of the light, her pain subsided almost instantly. Dinshah assumed it was because she was dying and had been released from further pain. He felt a flood of guilt as she turned her face to him and said: "Thank you for saving my life, Dinshah." But the woman knew from her internal bodily messages something that Dinshah did not know: She was not dying, but returning to life.

By late morning, Dinshah could see the improvement that his patient had already felt, hours before. Encouraged, he took a bottle of the same Indigo color from her kitchen, filled it with milk and placed it in the sun to absorb the magical energy that he was now convinced saved his patient's life. He fed this to his patient and her improvement accelerated.

Within 24 hours, Dinshah was astounded to see his patient sit up and demand food. By noon of that remarkable day, she was out of bed and taking a bath. He made a return visit the next day to be greeted by a radiant and admiring patient who was eager to tell the world about the amazing medical cure her young genius had devised. He made her promise not to tell anyone what he had done as he would be branded a quack and driven out of the "medical priesthood," as he called it.

This was the beginning of a 23-year quest for the healing power of light, culminating in a 1000-page book covering his research on the remarkable ability of various colors of light, externally applied, to heal an almost infinite variety of diseases.

Dinshah — "King of Duty"

Ghadiali spoke 18 languages and was naturalized an American citizen in 1917. He invented a flickerless motion picture machine, which may have been the first of its kind. He was appointed by the governor of New York as a colonel in the New York Police Air Service and flew the first police mail between New York and Philadelphia. For his meritorious service to the city of New York, he was awarded the Liberty Medal in 1919 by Mayor John Hylan.

But Dr. Ghadiali's attention was always drawn back to the light color therapy of his younger years in India. America, being the land of the free and not mired in a thousand years of conformity like India, was the perfect place, he thought, to continue his research on what he had come to call Spectro-Chrome. He formed the Spectro-Chrome Institute in New York and thus began a bitter struggle with the same dark forces that infect the medical faculty of every country in the world: an inexplicable desire to humiliate and destroy any innovative therapy that does not come from the halls of "acidemia." Any means, foul or fair, were used to destroy the miscreant, no matter what his qualifications or his reputation. He suffered more persecution in America than he ever would have in British colonial India.

He had to defend himself against law suits in Oregon, Ohio, Buffalo, Delaware, Washington D.C., Brooklyn, and twice in New Jersey. These suits were instituted by the states and the federal government, not by patients. He had spread knowledge of color therapy across the nation to natural healers and had to be stopped as an example to others who might step out of line.

In the Buffalo case, he was accused of "grand larceny" by the medical profession, backed by the state, because "Spectro-chrome could not possibly have any effect on disease." With lay and some professional witnesses testifying for him, he won the case. But when fighting a relentless enemy like established government, winning a case and establishing a "precedent" means nothing. His enemies had unlimited funds and kept after him relentlessly.

In Camden, New Jersey, they attempted to have him deported to India even though he had been a U.S. citizen for 17 years and was a decorated colonel and former commander of the New York Police Air Service. He avoided deportation after proving that he "was of the white race and therefore should not be deported"!

He lost all of the other cases, resulting in fines as high as $20,000 — the equivalent of a few hundred thousand dollars today — and served a total of 18 months in various American prisons. All this because he wanted doctors to try the simple expedient of treating patients with external, colored-light therapy.

His wife couldn't take the resulting depriva- tion and mental strain, deserted him and returned to India.

In 1941, his institute was hit with a "mail fraud order" by the U.S. Post Office. This ordered all postmasters across the country, with no hearing for the Spectro-Chrome Institute, to return to the sender all mail addressed to the "offender" stamped with the notation: *"Fraudulent,* Mail to this address returned by order of the Postmaster General."

A mysterious and devastating fire in 1945 destroyed the main building of the Institute, causing the loss of all of his scientific apparatus, other inventions, his library, medical case histories, and office equipment. The loss of the case histories seriously handicapped him in his defense in the Brooklyn lawsuit, which, conveniently for the government and the medical profession, came to trial only three months after the fire.

In 1947, a suit initiated by the Food and Drug Administration (FDA) resulted in a fine of $20,000, an order to dissolve the cursed Institute, and ordered him to dissociate himself from "any form of promotion of Spectro-Chrome." In a good old-fashioned book-burning, he was ordered to surrender for destruction $250,000 worth of books related to Spectro-Chrome. Like a common criminal, he was given "probation" which, if disobeyed, would put him back in jail.

Undaunted, in 1953, with the end of his probation, he organized another color therapy organization, the "Visible Spectrum Research Institute." This time the FDA, tired of fighting this pesky quack, obtained a permanent injunction through a federal judge, and finished him for good.

Thirty-five years later, and 30 years after Dinshah's death at the age of 89, the injunction still stands.

Dinshah means King of Duty — and certainly Ghadiali lived up to his given name. Although the medical profession and the government managed to squash this great man like a bug under a boot, they can't stop you and me from using the simple techniques he recommended, unless they can figure out how to outlaw all flashlights and color filters.

Chapter 2

The Nuts and Bolts of Color Therapy

Theatrical companies use plastic sheets of various colors, called color filters, to produce all those magical colored lights you see at musicals and other dramatic events. There's nothing complicated about it; they're just sheets of plastic, of specific colors, that are placed over the lights that beam down on the sets and performers to produce the dramatic effect needed for a particular scene.

These filters are what you need for self-treatment of everything from depression to diarrhea, from gas to gonorrhea, from headache to hemorrhoids, and from claustrophobia to chlorhistechia. There may be a little hyperbole there, but color therapy can *always* be used as an adjunct to traditional therapies — and your doctor doesn't even have to know about it. Let him have all the credit; doctors don't get many successes.

Another Unbelievable Story

Before I explain how you can do this simple treatment at home, let me tell you about the incredible case of little Grace Shirlow and then you will probably be as convinced as I am of the power of this simple treatment.

Eight-year-old Grace Shirlow was so badly burned that the surgeons had given up on her. Dr. Kate Baldwin, the senior surgeon at Women's Hospital in Philadelphia, Pennsylvania, took over the case. This great physician, contrary to all the medical knowledge of her time, and risking her career, became a disciple of Dinshah's color therapy. An abstract of Dr. Baldwin's article in the *Atlantic Medical Journal*, April 1927, is revealing and I strongly recommend that you read it (Please see Appendix). It is not esoteric verbiage, but simple enough for even a doctor to understand, although few of them have read it.

Grace's immediate problem was that she was about to die from anuria, the complete shutdown of her kidney function, which is common with severe burn cases. There had been almost complete cessation of urination for 48 hours. Death from anuria was hovering at her bedside. Dr. Baldwin applied the color Scarlet over the girl's kidneys at a distance of 18 inches. The rest of the body was shielded from the light. *Two hours later, she voided eight ounces of urine.*

Grace was treated with full-body Blue light after being snatched from death by the color Scarlet. Her pain immediately subsided and never returned. Her recovery was rapid and, in spite of severe third-degree burns, she had very little scarring.

Medicine Goes Backward

Today, almost 70 years later, we are further from the therapeutic use of light-color therapy than we were in the time of this great humanitarian and physician. Dr. Baldwin remarked to a colleague at the time that "I would close my office tonight never to reopen, if I could not use (color therapy)."

Remember that for every fool there is at least one heterodox medical idea. The trouble is that it's impossible to prove, or disprove, many of them. That's why quacks, as well as the gifted visionary, get persecuted equally by established medicine. Take electroacupuncture, for an example. Does it work to "adjust" the body and thus prevent disease? If the disease doesn't happen, then who knows what the treatment did, if anything. If the disease does happen, then you have proven that the treatment did not prevent the disease *in that particular case.*

But examples of orthodox blindness abound, scientific discoveries that obviously worked but were rejected by the science of the time. As far back as 1903, Scientific American was a very respected scientific publication; it still is. But in 1903, and for the following five years, *Scientific American* denied that the Wright brothers had flown a craft heavier than air. It was impossible, even though there were photographs and many public demonstrations of flights.

Thomas Edison, although his reputation as an inventor of genius proportions was well-established, was ridiculed and scorned by established science when he announced that he had invented an electric light. He demonstrated it on the streets, but scientists shunned the demonstrations as though they were from the devil himself. A prominent chemist named Henry Morton wrote that he felt "compelled to protest on behalf of true science. He said Edison's experiments were a conspicuous failure, trumpeted as a wonderful success."

Although it is abundantly clear that orthodox science is extremely narrow-minded and generally closed to new ideas, that does not mean that we should wholeheartedly endorse every crack-brained idea that comes along. In my opinion, color therapy long ago passed from the arena of the weird and the unproven into the field of a plausible and useful therapeutic method. It's just that most doctors don't know about it and, if they were told about it, would reject it out of hand.

This rejection phenomenon by medical science is a tragedy in the case of color therapy because it would cost practically nothing to prove or disprove it. If you treated a thousand cases of appendicitis, for example, with adjunctive light therapy (i.e., added to the traditional therapy), and the thousand so treated got well significantly quicker than those not receiving the light treatment, then the case would be proven.

Chapter 3

What It Is and How to Do It at Home

It's about time someone asked the question: "What in the world is happening with this color therapy? It's known that the red wavelength will penetrate the skin for a considerable distance, but it's also known that blue does not. How can blue then have any effect on the body's health?" Good question.

The idea of shining a specific color on a diseased part of the body for treatment will sound preposterous to most, but think about it: ultraviolet and infrared, both invisible parts of the electromagnetic spectrum, are readily recognized as useful in medicine, so why should anyone be surprised that the rest of the spectrum, i.e., visible light, is also useful? Applications of light, the color red, for instance, which has a frequency of 436,803,079,680,000 oscillations per second, is just as much a form of energy as the note high C, which has an oscillation frequency of 4,096 oscillations per second. X-rays, gamma-rays, delta-rays and magnetism are all forms of oscillatory energy. As far as we know, magnetism has the highest oscillatory rate, which is 18,446,744,073,709,551,616 oscillations per second. That's 18 quintillion, 446 quadrillion, 744 trillion, 73 billion, 709 million, 551 thousand, 6 hundred, and 16 oscillations per second. It is hard for the mind to grasp how anything can take place that many times in only one second. That's a long way from the oscillation of the lowest inaudible (to humans) sound, which is a mere two oscillations per second.

I'm dragging you through all of these numbers to help you understand colors which are not what you *see*, but what they *are*: vibratory energy. The average physician, unfamiliar with color therapy, would say: "That can't possibly have any effect – it's only color – it doesn't penetrate the skin." But what the average doctor doesn't realize is that the body, like all living things, has an electromagnetic field around it, and light therapy works very powerfully on the field. It does not have to penetrate the skin to have an effect.

With color therapy, what you see is not what you get (energy is very difficult to see). The color yellow, for instance, is 165 times brighter to the human eye than a lovely, gentle violet. While yellow has a brightness rating of 1,000, violet's rating is only six. Magenta, a very effective color for certain conditions, is even "weaker" as far as what you see is concerned, and is only one thousandth as bright as yellow. *What you see has nothing to do with the therapeutic effect* and every color has its place in the treatment of disease.

Color therapy is so simple, there's really no need to have doctors or clinics administering it. In fact, one of the reasons I like color therapy so much is that it helps you take your health into your own hands.

To do color therapy at home, all you need is a flashlight with fresh batteries, color filters (enclosed with this report), and a little patience. As far as the flashlight is concerned, don't go out and buy a 2000-watt blaster because you think that if the light from a four-cell flashlight is good, then the light from something the military might use to burn a hole through a tank will be better. Don't be concerned about the source of the light. Everything from sunlight to a pen light has been used successfully. Those square flashlights with a handle on them, about half the size of a loaf of bread, are as big a light as you will ever need for color therapy. *It's the quality of the light that generates the effect, not the quantity.* Remember that Dinshah treated his first dying patient with the light of a simple kerosene lantern.

I recommend you purchase a flashlight that has an adjustable beam, such as the Mag-Lite brand. These will allow you tonate (expose) your entire body or a specific region with the same flashlight. The only problem you may encounter with this type of flashlight is that they are round and may roll around when placed on a hard surface. But that's easily remedied by placing the flashlight on a pillow.

While Mag-Lites come in several different sizes, I recommend that you purchase the largest size. The smaller pocket-sized lights will work for tonations on specific regions, but I've found their beam to be too small for whole-body tonations. When you expand the beam on the larger sizes, you'll notice the beam is most concentrated in the middle and is weaker around the edges. Don't worry about that. Remember, it's quality, not quantity, that we want.

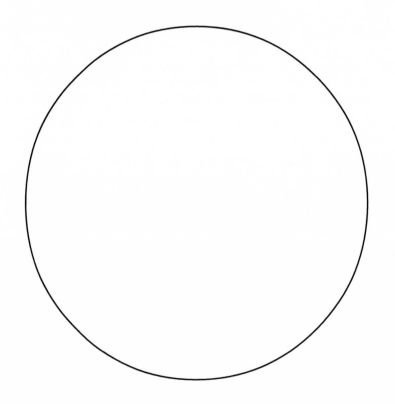

Make sure that whatever brand or style of flashlight you buy, the lens is no bigger than four inches in diameter. If your flashlight lens is bigger than the circle on the preceding page, you'll have to find a smaller flashlight in order to use the enclosed filters. (The Mag-Lites lenses on the larger sizes are only about two inches in diameter.)

In the past, people have found that mounting the plastic filters in front of the light is difficult. Some patients have fashioned an attachment out of a coat hanger. But we have found an even easier way, which we will explain in a moment. Actually, Ghadiali had the perfect instruments for all this, but the government smashed them all with a sledgehammer — for your protection, of course.

The filters we ye enclosed with this report are four-inch squares. On most flashlights, the plastic lens unscrews from the front of your flashlight. Using the lens as a pattern, cut the filter to the same size with an X-acto knife or scissors (the X-acto knife will work the best, but make sure you place a pile of old newspapers under the filter so you don't damage your table — and be careful, these knives are extremely sharp). Take special care not to tear or cut into the circle; you want as clean of a cut as you can get. Place the filter on top of the lens and reassemble the flashlight. When you turn the flashlight on, you should see only colored light. If you do, then you know you've done it correctly.

If you decide to use a lamp instead of a flashlight, make sure you don't place the filter too close to the light (placing it several inches away may be required).

Many lamps can be very hot and will burn the filter. If you use a cool fluorescent lamp, burning will not be a problem. If you find the four-inch filters to be too small, please call Rhino Publishing at 1-888-317-6767 or 416-352-5126. They can help you order filters as large as 20″ x 24″. (It takes two and a half filters of this size to cover the average ceiling fluorescent light.)

General Guidelines

It's important to use the exact colors that Dinshah recommended. That is, if Indigo is recommended, don't use Blue or Violet. If one isn't working as it is supposed to, either you and your doctor have the wrong diagnosis or some other color, or color combination, is required. Try something else; you're not going to kill yourself, and you'll be fine as long as you're otherwise getting good basic medical advice. What you are doing is in addition to what the doctor has prescribed, not counter to it.

A tonation (exposure) with a specific color is usually done for one hour. You may want to tonate the front and back. For something specific, like an ulcer on the leg, there is no need to tonate anything but the affected area.

Put the light source six to 18 inches from the affected area. For whole-body tonation, that is not possible and you will have to settle for whatever distance it takes to cover the entire body, depending on your light mechanism. For specific lesions, again using the ulcer example, you can concentrate the tonation by placing shades around the light source (if you're not using an adjustable beam flashlight).

The room does not have to be completely dark, but definitely on the shady side. Competing direct light, from a lamp or sun rays through a window, for instance, will destroy the effects of the tonation. When I was doing photo-oxidation therapy, requiring an intravenous drip, we tried to do concurrent color treatment. It was not successful because the nurses had to observe the patients practically constantly and the lack of light made them feel uneasy about the possibility of missing something. We set aside one area as a "dark room," to teach patients how to use the therapy, then they applied it at home. This worked very well.

Chapter 4

Specific Colors

What you have read here is a simplification of the color therapy process. I am going to give you some easy-to-use, at-home color treatments for certain problems that, although not life-threatening, are fraught with trauma to your system and to your pocketbook.

You'll notice the filters you have purchased each has a number. These numbers will help you create the proper colors for your specific ailment. (After cutting the filters, make sure you keep track of the number. You'll need to know which filter goes with each number. I recommend labeling the cut-out portion of the filter with a black, fine-point, permanent marker. (If you get your filters from a professional art studio or stage outlet, they will be numbered according to the color.)

Get the following filters:

Yellow	809
Gold	810
Cherry	818

Pink	826
Grape	828
Fuschsia	832
Lt. Blue	859
Med. Blue	861
Dark Blue	866 (this is Dinshah's Blue)
Green	871
Teal	877

Creating many of the Dinshah colors requires placing two or three filters on your flashlight at the same time. To create the color specified, assemble the filters in the following manner:

Red	818, 828
Yellow	809
Green	871
Blue	866
Violet	832, 859, 866
Magenta	818, 828, 866
Orange	809, 828
Lemon	809, 871
Turquoise	861, 871
Indigo	832, 877
Purple	832, 866
Scarlet	810, 818, 861

You can also create "in-between" colors if you find that one of the above colors is too strong or too weak. If, for instance, you find that Orange is too powerful for your particular case, and Yellow might not be strong enough, you can try an in-between color.

Red-Orange	809, 818
Lemon-Green	810, 871
Turquoise-Blue	871, 866
Orange-Yellow	809, 826
Green-Turquoise	871, 877

Chapter 5

Specific Ailments

Some of the ailments listed below call for some colors to be used systemically. All that means is to expose the entire body with that particular color.

<u>This is very important, because without an hour of the full-body tonation, many of the treatments will not work.</u>

Abscesses — Tonate Indigo to the affected area. May need surgical incision followed by tonation.

Angina (chest pain beneath the breast bone) — Lemon and Magenta systemic front (entire length of the body) for prophylaxis. Purple over the upper chest during an attack. Have an exam by a "competent physician" i.e., a doctor who practices cardiology.

Arrhythmia (irregular heart beat) — Lemon or Magenta, systemic front.

Arthritis — *Acute*: Green systemic then Indigo to affected area. *Chronic*: Lemon systemic then Indigo to affected area.

Asthma — *During* an attack: Purple on face, neck, and upper chest. If not effective, switch to

Orange. Scarlet on lower back (take tonation on side and not lying on the stomach). *Between attacks:* Lemon systemic front, followed by Orange on front of neck and upper chest.

Boils — Lemon systemic, then Orange to affected area until suppuration (draining) starts, then switch to Violet.

Bronchitis — Turquoise systemic front, then Violet or Purple to face, neck, and upper chest (breast area).

Bruises — Indigo to affected area as soon as possible. After the pain subsides, Orange to affected area.

Burns — Indigo to affected area; may need extended tonation if severe. After the pain subsides, use Turquoise systemic and then Green to affected area.

Cataract — Lemon systemic front then Magenta on upper chest. This is for prevention and arresting an early cataract. It is not effective for mature cataracts.

Colds — Green systemic front followed by Blue on face and neck.

Constipation — Lemon systemic front followed by Yellow to the abdomen and pelvis. If the condition does not respond, switch to Orange.

Diabetes — Lemon systemic front then Yellow to entire abdomen. Insulin requirements may be reduced. Seek the treatment of an endocrinologist.

Diarrhea — Yellow on entire abdomen once, then Turquoise systemic front. If Yellow is not effective in 24 hours, switch to Indigo.

Drowsiness, chronic — Lemon systemic followed by Magenta systemic, front and back (tonate the black while lying on the side). Scarlet may be used if the blood pressure is not elevated.

Earache — Turquoise systemic front followed by Orange to affected area. If there is an infection, heat and antibiotics may be needed. -- see a physician.

Flu — Same as for colds.

Gastroenteritis (colitis, "dysentery") — Green systemic to the front of the body followed by Yellow to the entire abdomen and pelvis for two tonations, then Indigo to the same area.

Hair loss — Lemon systemic front followed by Orange to area of hair loss.

Hay fever (respiratory allergy) — Lemon systemic front then Turquoise or Blue to face.

Headache — Purple to face and upper chest (breast area).

Heartburn — Green systemic front then Blue on neck and upper chest.

Hiccup — Orange on abdomen above hip bones and Indigo to back of neck.

Impotence — Green systemic front and then Scarlet to genital area.

Indigestion — Orange on lower chest, and entire abdomen.

Insomnia — Violet to face.

Menstrual cramps — Orange to genital area and lower abdomen. Scarlet to lower back while lying on side.

Muscle cramps — Orange to affected area.

Nausea — Orange on lower chest and upper abdomen.

Obesity — As an appetite suppressant: Lemon systemic front followed by Violet over the entire abdomen.

Prostate enlargement (benign prostatic hypertrophy) — Lemon systemic front followed by Orange and/or Indigo at the lower back (lying on side) and at the genital area. There are other effective treatments which can be used concurrently such has saw palmetto. Get examined by a urologist.

Shingles — Acute: Green systemic followed by Indigo to affected area. Chronic: Violet to painful area.

Sinus inflammation (sinusitis) —Green systemic followed by Blue to the face.

Skin conditions — Moist: Turquoise systemic until signs of drying, then Indigo to affected area. Thy or scaly: Lemon systemic daily followed by Orange to affected area until it begins to weep, then go to Indigo.

Sore throat — Green systemic to front of body then Blue to face and neck. If the condition persists or worsens, see a physician.

Sprains — Indigo to affected area.

****

To increase the effectiveness of the treatment even further, or as an alternative treatment when tonation is not practical, water can be color-charged. Using a glass container, (pure crystal glass is best), expose the water to the desired color for at least an hour then drink it. For a "broad-spectrum" therapy, expose water to sunlight. When doing so, use pure crystal glass or the water will not be properly energized.

Some caveats:

* Many localized conditions will not respond until systemic (full body) tonation is done.

* Each tonation procedure should be for one hour.

* If the condition is severe, tonation can be given continuously.

* Avoid treatment during menses, if possible.

* Never tonate the back from a prone (on the abdomen) position — always on the side. All tonations otherwise can be done while lying on the back and this position is preferred. So always lie face-up or on the side — never lie face down. For reasons not yet known, color therapy does not work if you lie on your stomach.

* The room should be in at least semi-darkness. Avoid competing light from windows or lamps. Total darkness is not necessary.

* The tonating room should be warm for best results — the warmer the better.

* It is best not to read or watch television during treatment, especially during systemic (whole-body) tonation. Learn to sleep or day dream during treatment

* All tonation should be applied directly to the skin and at a distance of not more than 18 inches, except for systemic applications.

* The darker colors, such as Indigo, are not easily seen on the skin, but don't let this concern you. What you see is not what you get.

* Except when using color therapy as a digestive aid, allow one hour between eating and tonating.

* Use only one method of healing at a time if you can. If using drugs in conjunction with color therapy, interactions are possible although not common.

* Due to their cleansing effect, a rash or diarrhea may occur when first using Lemon, Green, or Turquoise.

* When in doubt, start with Green systemic front. Green is the middle color in the spectrum and has a balancing effect.

* In extremely old or debilitated persons, color therapy may be ineffective. There are limitations to all therapies and death can not be averted forever.

Conclusion

Now that you've read a little bit about this remarkable treatment, go ahead and try it for yourself. You'll soon see that color therapy is truly remarkable, if done properly.

Color therapy has been around longer than most modern medical treatments and is more effective than many of them (it's certainly safer). It's truly a shame that this therapy has been suppressed all these years. But the treatment has survived and even flourished in some parts of the world. Maybe now it will flourish in the United States.

If you would like a more detailed exposition on color therapy, please read either the 1000-page treatise, Spectro-Chrome Metry Encyclopedia, or the condensed version by Ghadiali's son, Darius Dinshah, entitled Let There Be Light available from the Dinshah Health Society at www.dinshahhealth.org

Appendix

The Therapeutic Value of Light and Color

Kate W. Baldwin, M.D., F.A.C.S.

In the effort to obtain relief from suffering, many of the more simple but potent measures have been overlooked while we have grasped at the obscure and complicated.

Sunlight is the basic source of all life and energy upon earth. Deprive plant or animal life of light, and it soon shows the lack and ceases to develop. Place a seed in the very best of soil or a human being in a palace, shut out the light and what happens? Without food (in the usual sense of the term) man can live many days; without liquids a much shorter time; but not at all without the atmosphere which surrounds him at all times and to which he pays so little attention. The forces upon which life mostly depends are placed nearly, or quite beyond, personal control.

For centuries, scientists have devoted untiring effort to discover means for the relief or cure of human ills and restoration of the normal functions. Yet, in neglected light and color, there is a potency far beyond that of drugs and serums.

In order that the whole body may function perfectly, each organ must be 100 percent perfect. When the spleen, the liver, or any other organ falls below normal, it simply means that the body laboratories have not provided the required materials with which to work, either because they are not functioning as a result of some disorder of the internal mechanism, or because they have not been provided with the necessary materials. Before the body can appropriate the required elements, they must be separated from the waste matter.

Each element gives off a characteristic color wave. The prevailing color wave of hydrogen is red and that of oxygen is blue, and each element in turn gives off its own special color wave. Sunlight, as it is received by the body, is split into the prismatic colors and their combinations as white light is split by passage through a prism. Everything on the red side of the spectrum is more or less stimulating, while the blue is sedative. There are many shades of each color and each is produced by a little different wave length. Just as sound waves are tuned to each other and produce harmony or discords, so color waves may be tuned and only so can they be depended on always to produce the same results.

If one requires a dose of castor oil, he does not go to a drug store and request a little portion from each bottle on the shelves. I see no virtue, then, in the use of the whole white light as a therapeutic measure when the different colors can give what is required without taxing the body to rid itself of that for which it has no use, and which may do more or less harm. If the body is sick it should be restored with the least possible effort. There is no more accurate or easier way than by giving the color representing the lacking elements, and the body will, through its radioactive forces, appropriate them and so restore the normal balance. *Color is the simplest and most accurate therapeutic measure yet developed.*

For about six years, I have given close attention to the action of colors in restoring the body functions, and I am perfectly honest in saying that, after nearly 37 years of active hospital and private practice in medicine and surgery, I can produce quicker and more accurate results with colors than with any or all other methods combined — and with less strain on the patient. In many cases, the functions have been restored after the classical remedies have failed. Of course, surgery is necessary in some cases, but the results will be quicker and better if color is used before and after the operation. Sprains, bruises, and traumata of all sorts respond to color as to no other treatment.

Septic conditions yield, regardless of the specific organism. Cardiac lesions, asthma, hay fever, pneumonia, inflammatory conditions of the eyes, corneal ulcers, and cataracts are relieved by the treatment.

The treatment of carbuncles (large and deep sores of the skin) with color is easy, compared to the classic methods. One woman with a carbuncle involving the back of the neck, from mastoid to mastoid (from ear to ear) and from occipital ridge to the first dorsal vertebra (the entire length of the neck), came under color therapy after ten days of the very best of attention. From the first day of color application, no opiates, not even sedatives, were required. This patient was saved much suffering and she has little scarring.

The use of color in the treatment of burns is well worth investigating by every member of the profession. In such cases, the burning sensation caused by the destructive forces may be counteracted in from 20 to 30 minutes, and it does not return. True burns are caused by the destructive action of the red side of the spectrum, hydrogen predominating. Apply oxygen by the use of the blue side of the spectrum and much will be done to relieve the nervous strain, the healing processes are rapid, and the resulting tissues soft and flexible.

In very extensive burns in a child of eight years of age, there was almost complete suppression of urine for more than 48 hours with a temperature of 105 to 106 degrees. Fluids were forced to no effect and a more hopeless case is seldom seen. Scarlet was applied just over the kidneys at a distance of 18 inches for 20 minutes, all other areas being covered. Two hours later, the child voided eight ounces of urine.

In some unusual and extreme cases that had not responded to other treatment, normal functioning has been restored by color therapy. At present, therefore, I do not feel justified in refusing any case without a trial. Even in cases where death is inevitable, much comfort may be secured.

There is no question that light and color are important therapeutic media and that their adoption will be of advantage to both the profession and the people. (Emphasis was added.)

Atlantic Medical Journal, April 1927.

Note: This remarkable report is as authentic and useful as it was 75 years ago! -- William Campbell Douglass, MD

About Doctor William Campbell Douglass II

Dr. Douglass reveals medical truths, and deceptions, often at risk of being labeled heretical. He is consumed by a passion for living a long healthy life, and wants his readers to share that passion. Their health and well-being comes first. He is anti-dogmatic, and unwavering in his dedication to improve the quality of life of his readers. He has been called "the conscience of modern medicine," a "medical maverick," and has been voted "Doctor of the Year" by the National Health Federation. His medical experiences are far reaching-from battling malaria in Central America - to fighting deadly epidemics at his own health clinic in Africa - to flying with U.S. Navy crews as a flight surgeon - to working for 10 years in emergency medicine here in the States. These learning experiences, not to mention his keen storytelling ability and wit, make Dr. Douglass' newsletters (Daily Dose and Real Health) and books uniquely interesting and fun to read. He shares his no-frills, no-bull approach to health care, often amazing his readers by telling them to ignore many widely-hyped good-health practices (like staying away from red meat, avoiding coffee, and eating like a bird), and start living again by eating REAL food, taking some inexpensive supplements, and doing the pleasurable things that make life livable. Readers get all this, plus they learn how to burn fat, prevent cancer, boost libido, and so much more. And, Dr. Douglass is not afraid to challenge the latest studies that come out, and share the real story with his readers. Dr. William C. Douglass has led a colorful, rebellious, and crusading life. Not many physicians would dare put their professional reputations on the line as many times as this courageous healer has. A vocal opponent of "business-as-usual" medicine, Dr. Douglass has championed patients' rights and physician commitment to wellness throughout his career. This dedicated physician has repeatedly gone far beyond the call of duty in his work to spread the truth about alternative therapies. For a full year, he endured economic and physical hardship to work with physicians at the Pasteur Institute in St. Petersburg, Russia, where advanced research on photoluminescence was being conducted. Dr. Douglass comes from a distinguished family of physicians. He is the fourth generation Douglass to practice medicine, and his son is also a physician. Dr. Douglass graduated from the University of Rochester, the Miami School of Medicine, and the Naval School of Aviation and Space Medicine.

You want to protect those you love from the health dangers the authorities aren't telling you about, and learn the incredible cures that they've scorned and ignored?
Subscribe to the free Daily Dose updates "...the straight scoop about health, medicine, and politics." by sending an e-mail to real_sub@agoramail.net with the word "subscribe" in the subject line.

Dr. William Campbell Douglass'
Real Health:

Had Enough?

Enough turkey burgers and sprouts?

Enough forcing gallons of water down your throat?

Enough exercising until you can barely breathe?

Before you give up everything just because "everyone" says it's healthy...

Learn the facts from Dr. William Campbell Douglass, medicine's most acclaimed myth-buster. In every issue of Dr. Douglass' Real Health newsletter, you'll learn shocking truths about "junk medicine" and how to stay healthy while eating eggs, meat and other foods you love.

With the tips you'll receive from Real Health, you'll see your doctor less, spend a lot less money and be happier and healthier while you're at it. The road to Real Health is actually easier, cheaper and more pleasant than you dared to dream.

Subscribe to Real Health today by calling 1-800-981-7162 or visit the Real Health web site at www.realhealthnews.com.
Use promotional code : DRHBDZZZ

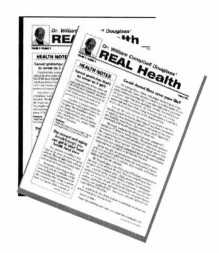

If you knew of a procedure that could save thousands, maybe millions, of people dying from AIDS, cancer, and other dreaded killers....

Would you cover it up?

It's unthinkable that what could be the best solution ever to stopping the world's killer diseases is being ignored, scorned, and rejected. But that is exactly what's happening right now.

The procedure is called "photoluminescence". It's a thoroughly tested, proven therapy that uses the healing power of the light to perform almost miraculous cures.

This remarkable treatment works its incredible cures by stimulating the body's own immune responses. That's why it cures so many ailments--and why it's been especially effective against AIDS! Yet, 50 years ago, it virtually disappeared from the halls of medicine.

Why has this incredible cure been ignored by the medical authorities of this country? You'll find the shocking answer here in the pages of this new edition of Into the Light. Now available with the blood irradiation Instrument Diagram and a complete set of instructions for building your own "Treatment Device". Also includes details on how to use this unique medical instrument.

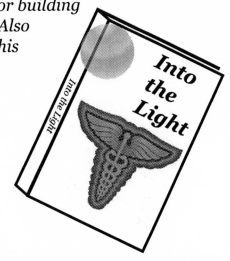

Rhino Publishing S.A.
www.rhinopublish.com

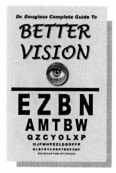

Dr. Douglass' Complete Guide to Better Vision

A report about eyesight and what can be done to improve it naturally. But I've also included information about how the eye works, brief descriptions of various common eye conditions, traditional remedies to eye problems, and a few simple suggestions that may help you maintain your eyesight for years to come.
-William Campbell Douglass II, MD

The Hypertension Report.
Say Good Bye to High Blood Pressure.

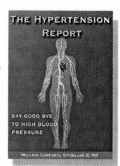

An estimated 50 million Americans have high blood pressure. Often called the "silent killer" because it may not cause symptoms until the patient has suffered serious damage to the arterial system. Diet, exercise, potassium supplements chelation therapy and practically anything but drugs is the way to go and alternatives are discussed in this report.

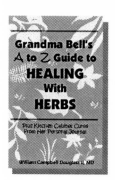

Grandma Bell's A To Z Guide To Healing With Herbs.

This book is all about - coming home. What I once believed to be old wives' tales - stories long destroyed by the new world of science - actually proved to be the best treatment for many of the common ailments you and I suffer through. So I put a few of them together in this book with the sincere hope that Grandma Bell's wisdom will help you recover your common sense, and take responsibility for your own health. -William Campbell Douglass II, MD

Prostate Problems:
Safe, Simple, Effective Relief for Men over 50.

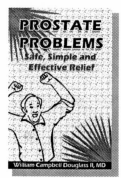

Don't be frightened into surgery or drugs you may not need. First, get the facts about prostate problems... know all your options, so you can make the best decisions. This fully documented report explains the dangers of conventional treatments, and gives you alternatives that could save you more than just money!

What Is Going on Here?

Peroxides are supposed to be bad for you. Free radicals and all that. But now we hear that hydrogen peroxide is good for us. Hydrogen peroxide will put extra oxygen in your blood. There's no doubt about that. Hydrogen peroxide costs pennies. So if you can get oxygen into the blood cheaply and safely, maybe cancer (which doesn't like oxygen), emphysema, AIDS, and many other terrible diseases can be treated effectively. Intravenous hydrogen peroxide rapidly relieves allergic reactions, influenza symptoms, and acute viral infections.

No one expects to live forever. But we would all like to have a George Burns finish. The prospect of finishing life in a nursing home after abandoning your tricycle in the mobile home park is not appealing. Then comes the loss of control of vital functions the ultimate humiliation. Is life supposed to be from tricycle to tricycle and diaper to diaper? You come into this world crying, but do you have to leave crying? I don't believe you do. And you won't either after you see the evidence. Sounds too good to be true, doesn't it? Read on and decide for yourself.

-William Campbell Douglass II, MD

Rhino Publishing S.A.
www.rhinopublish.com

HYDROGEN PEROXIDE

Medical Miracle

H_2O

Don't drink your milk!

If you knew what we know about milk... BLEECHT! All that pasteurization, homogenization and processing is not only cooking all the nutrients right out of your favorite drink. It's also adding toxic levels of vitamin D.

This fascinating book tells the whole story about milk. How it once was nature's perfect food...how "raw," unprocessed milk can heal and boost your immune system ... why you can't buy it legally in this country anymore, and what we could do to change that.

Dr. "Douglass traveled all over the world, tasting all kinds of milk from all kinds of cows, poring over dusty research books in ancient libraries far from home, to write this light-hearted but scientifically sound book.

Rhino Publishing, S.A.
www.rhinopublish.com

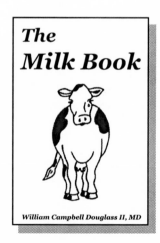

The Milk Book

William Campbell Douglass II, MD

Eat Your Cholesterol!

Eat Meat, Drink Milk, Spread The Butter- And Live Longer!
How to Live off the Fat of the Land and Feel Great.

Americans are being saturated with anti-cholesterol propaganda. If you watch very much television, you're probably one of the millions of Americans who now has a terminal case of cholesterol phobia. The propaganda is relentless and is often designed to produce fear and loathing of this worst of all food contaminants. You never hear the food propagandists bragging about their product being fluoride-free or aluminum-free, two of our truly serious food-additive problems. But cholesterol, an essential nutrient, not proven to be harmful in any quantity, is constantly pilloried as a menace to your health. If you don't use corn oil, Fleischmann's margarine, and Egg Beaters, you're going straight to atherosclerosis hell with stroke, heart attack, and premature aging -- and so are your kids. Never feel guilty about what you eat again! Dr. Douglass shows you why red meat, eggs, and dairy products aren't the dietary demons we're told they are. But beware: This scientifically sound report goes against all the "common wisdom" about the foods you should eat. Read with an open mind.

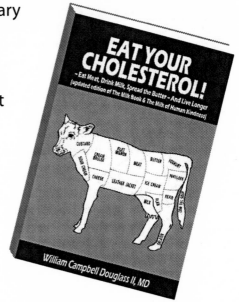

Rhino Publishing, S.A.
www.rhinopublish.com

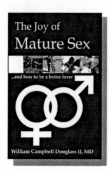

The Joy of Mature Sex and How to Be a Better Lover

Humans are very confused about what makes good sex. But I believe humans have more to offer each other than this total licentiousness common among animals. We're talking about mature sex. The kind of sex that made this country great.

Stop Aging or Slow the Process How Exercise With Oxygen Therapy (EWOT) Can Help

EWOT (pronounced ee-watt) stands for Exercise With Oxygen Therapy. This method of prolonging your life is so simple and you can do it at home at a minimal cost. When your cells don't get enough oxygen, they degenerate and die and so you degenerate and die. It's as simple as that.

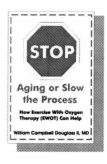

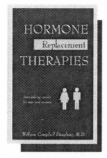

Hormone Replacement Therapies: Astonishing Results For Men And Women

It is accurate to say that when the endocrine glands start to fail, you start to die. We are facing a sea change in longevity and health in the elderly. Now, with the proper supplemental hormones, we can slow the aging process and, in many cases, reverse some of the signs and symptoms of aging.

Add 10 Years to Your Life With some "best of" Dr. Douglass' writings.

To add ten years to your life, you need to have the right attitude about health and an understanding of the health industry and what it's feeding you. Following the established line on many health issues could make you very sick or worse! Achieve dynamic health with this collection of some of the "best of" Dr. Douglass' newsletters.

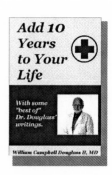

How did AIDS become one of the Greatest Biological Disasters in the History of Mankind?

GET THE FACTS

AIDS and BIOLOGICAL WARFARE covers the history of plagues from the past to today's global confrontation with AIDS, the Prince of Plagues. Completely documented *AIDS and BIOLOGICAL WARFARE* helps you make your own decisions about how to survive in a world ravaged by this horrible plague.

You will learn that AIDS is not a naturally occuring disease process as you have been led to believe, but a man-made biological nightmare that has been unleashed and is now threatening the very existence of human life on the planet.

There is a smokescreen of misinformation clouding the AIDS issue. Now, for the first time, learn the truth about the nature of the crisis our planet faces: its origin -- how AIDS is really transmited and alternatives for treatment. Find out what they are not telling you about AIDS and Biological Warfare, and how to protect yourself and your loved ones. AIDS is a serious problem worldwide, but it is no longer the major threat. You need to know the whole story. To protect yourself, you must know the truth about biological warfare.

PAINFUL DILEMMA

Are we fighting the wrong war?

We are spending millions on the war against drugs while we
should be fighting the war against pain with those drugs!

As you will read in this book, the war on drugs was lost a long time ago and,
when it comes to the war against pain, pain is winning! An article in USA Today
(11/20/02) reveals that dying patients are not getting relief from pain. It seems
the doctors are torn between fear of the government, certainly justified, and a
clinging to old and out dated ideas about pain, which is NOT justified.

A group called Last Acts, a coalition of health-care groups, has released a very
discouraging study of all 50 states that nearly half of the 1.6 million Americans
living in nursing homes suffer from untreated pain. They said that life was being
extended but it amounted to little more than "extended pain and suffering."

This book offers insight into the history of pain treatment and the current failed
philosophies of contemporary medicine. Plus it describes some of today's most
advanced treatments for alleviating certain kinds of pain. This book is not another
"self-help" book touting home remedies; rather, Painful Dilemma: Patients in
Pain -- People in Prison, takes a hard look at where we've gone wrong and what
we (you) can do to help a loved one who is living with chronic pain.

The second half of this book is a must read if you value your freedom. We now
have the ridiculous and tragic situation of people
in pain living in a government-created hell by
restriction of narcotics and people in prison for
trying to bring pain relief by the selling of
narcotics to the suffering. The end result of the
"war on drugs" has been to create the greatest
and most destructive cartel in history, so great,
in fact, that the drug Mafia now controls most
of the world economy.

Rhino Publishing S.A.
www.rhinopublish.com

Live the Adventure!

Why would anyone in their right mind put everything they own in storage and move to Russia, of all places?! But when maverick physician Bill Douglass left a profitable medical practice in a peaceful mountaintop town to pursue "pure medical truth".... none of us who know him well was really surprised.

After All, anyone who's braved the outermost reaches of darkest Africa, the mean streets of Johannesburg and New York, and even a trip to Washington to testify before the Senate, wouldn't bat and eye at ducking behind the Iron Curtain for a little medical reconnaissance!

Enjoy this imaginative, funny, dedicated man's tales of wonder and woe as he treks through a year in St. Petersburg, working on a cure for the world's killer diseases. We promise --

YOU WON'T BE BORED!

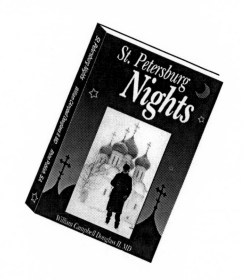

Rhino Publishing S.A.
www.rhinopublish.com

THE SMOKER'S PARADOX
THE HEALTH BENEFITS OF TOBACCO!

The benefits of smoking tobacco have been common knowledge for centuries. From sharpening mental acuity to maintaining optimal weight, the relatively small risks of smoking have always been outweighed by the substantial improvement to mental and physical health. Hysterical attacks on tobacco notwithstanding, smokers always weigh the good against the bad and puff away or quit according to their personal preferences. Now the same anti-tobacco enterprise that has spent billions demonizing the pleasure of smoking is providing additional reasons to smoke. Alzheimer's, Parkinson's, Tourette's Syndrome, even schizophrenia and cocaine addiction are disorders that are alleviated by tobacco. Add in the still inconclusive indication that tobacco helps to prevent colon and prostate cancer and the endorsement for smoking tobacco by the medical establishment is good news for smokers and non-smokers alike. Of course the revelation that tobacco is good for you is ruined by the pharmaceutical industry's plan to substitute the natural and relatively inexpensive tobacco plant with their overpriced and ineffective nicotine substitutions. Still, when all is said and done, the positive revelations regarding tobacco are very good reasons indeed to keep lighting those cigars - but only 4 a day!

Rhino Publishing, S.A
www.rhinopublish.com

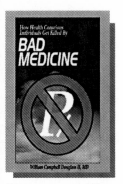

Bad Medicine
How Individuals Get Killed By Bad Medicine.

Do you really need that new prescription or that overnight stay in the hospital? In this report, Dr. Douglass reveals the common medical practices and misconceptions endangering your health. Best of all, he tells you the pointed (but very revealing!) questions your doctor prays you never ask. Interesting medical facts about popular remedies are revealed.

Dangerous Legal Drugs
The Poisons in Your Medicine Chest.

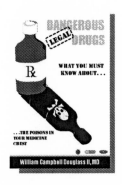

If you knew what we know about the most popular prescription and over-the-counter drugs, you'd be sick. That's why Dr. Douglass wrote this shocking report about the poisons in your medicine chest. He gives you the low-down on different categories of drugs. Everything from painkillers and cold remedies to tranquilizers and powerful cancer drugs.

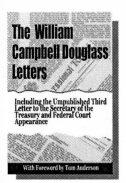

The William Campbell Douglass Letters.
Expose of Government Machinations (Vietnam War).

THE WILLIAM CAMPBELL DOUGLASS LETTERS. Dr. Douglass' Defense in 1968 Tax Case and Expose of Government Machinations during the Vietnam War.

The Eagle's Feather. A Novel of International Political Intrigue.

Although The Eagle's Feather is a work of fiction set in the 1970's, it is built, as with most fiction, on a framework of plausibility and background information. This is a fiction book that could not have been written were it not for various ominous aspects, which pose a clear and present danger to the security of the United States.

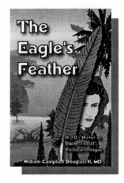

Rhino Publishing 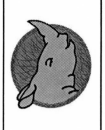	ORDER FORM

PURCHASER INFORMATION

Purchaser's Name (Please Print): _____

Shipping Address (Do not use a P.O. Box): _____

City: _____ State/Prov.: _____ Country: _____

Zip/Postal Code: _____ Telephone No.: _____ Fax No.: _____

E-Mail Address (if interested in receiving free e-Books when available): _____

CREDIT CARD INFO (CIRCLE ONE):

MASTERCARD, VISA, AMERICAN EXPRESS, DISCOVER, JCB, DINER'S CLUB, CARTE BLANCHE.

Charge my Card -> Number #: _____ Exp.: _____

*Security Code: _____ * Required for all MasterCard, Visa and American Express purchases. For your security, we require that you enter your card's verification number. The verification number is also called a CCV number. This code is the 3 digits farthest right in the signature field on the back of your VISA/MC, or the 4 digits to the right on the front of your American Express card. Your credit card statement will show **a different name than Rhino Publishing** as the vendor.

WE DO NOT share your private information, we use 3rd party credit card processing service to process your order only.

ADDITIONAL INFORMATION

If your shipping address is not the same as your credit card billing address, please indicate your card billing address here.

_____   Type of card: _____
Name on the card

Billing Address: _____

City: _____   State/Prov.: _____   Zip/Postal Code: _____

Fax a copy of this order to:
RHINO PUBLISHING, S.A.
1-888-317-6767 or International #: + 416-352-5126

To order by mail, send your payment by first class mail only to the following address. Please include a copy of this order form. Make your check or bank drafts (NO postal money order) payable to RHINO PUBLISHING, S.A. and mail to:

Rhino Publishing, S.A.
Attention: PTY 5048
P.O. Box 025724
Miami, FL.
USA 33102

Digital E-books also available online: www.rhinopublish.com

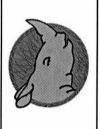

Rhino Publishing

ORDER FORM

Purchaser's Name (Please Print):

I would like to order the following paperback book of Dr. Douglass (Alternative Medicine Books):

___	X	9962-636-04-3	Add 10 Years to Your Life. With some "best of" Dr. Douglass writings.	$13.99 $ ___
___	X	9962-636-07-8	AIDS and Biological Warfare. What They Are Not Telling You!	$17.99 $ ___
___	X	9962-636-09-4	Bad Medicine. How Individuals Get Killed By Bad Medicine.	$11.99 $ ___
___	X	9962-636-10-8	Color Me Healthy. The Healing Power of Colors.	$11.99 $ ___
___	X	9962-636 -XX-X	Color Filters for Color Me Healthy. 11 Basic Roscolene Filters for Lamps.	$21.89 $ ___
___	X	9962-636-15-9	Dangerous Legal Drugs. The Poisons in Your Medicine Chest.	$13.99 $ ___
___	X	9962-636-18-3	Dr. Douglass' Complete Guide to Better Vision. Improve eyesight naturally.	$11.99 $ ___
___	X	9962-636-19-1	Eat Your Cholesterol! How to Live off the Fat of the Land and Feel Great.	$11.99 $ ___
___	X	9962-636-12-4	Grandma Bell's A To Z Guide To Healing. Her Kitchen Cabinet Cures.	$14.99 $ ___
___	X	9962-636-22-1	Hormone Replacement Therapies. Astonishing Results For Men & Women	$11.99 $ ___
___	X	9962-636-25-6	Hydrogen Peroxide: One of the Most Underused Medical Miracle.	$15.99 $ ___
___	X	9962-636-27-2	Into the Light. New Edition with Blood Irradiation Instrument Instructions.	$19.99 $ ___
___	X	9962-636-54-X	Milk Book. The Classic on the Nutrition of Milk and How to Benefit from it.	$17.99 $ ___

___	X	9962-636-00-0	Painful Dilemma - Patients in Pain - People in Prison.	$17.99	$ ___
___	X	9962-636-32-9	Prostate Problems. Safe, Simple, Effective Relief for Men over 50.	$11.99	$ ___
___	X	9962-636-34-5	St. Petersburg Nights. Enlightening Story of Life and Science in Russia.	$17.99	$ ___
___	X	9962-636-37-X	Stop Aging or Slow the Process. Exercise With Oxygen Therapy Can Help.	$11.99	$ ___
___	X	9962-636-60-4	The Hypertension Report. Say Good Bye to High Blood Pressure.	$11.99	$ ___
___	X	9962-636-48-5	The Joy of Mature Sex and How to Be a Better Lover...	$13.99	$ ___
___	X	9962-636-43-4	The Smoker's Paradox: Health Benefits of Tobacco.	$14.99	$ ___

Political Books:

___	X	9962-636-40-X	The Eagle's Feather. A 70's Novel of International Political Intrigue.	$15.99	$ ___
___	X	9962-636-46-9	The W. C. D. Letters. Expose of Government Machinations (Vietnam War).	$11.99	$ ___

SUB-TOTAL: $ ___

ADD $5.00 HANDLING FOR YOUR ORDER: $ 5.00 $ 5.00

___ X ADD $2.50 SHIPPING FOR EACH ITEM ON ORDER: $ 2.50 $ ___

NOTE THAT THE MINIMUM SHIPPING AND HANDLING IS $7.50 FOR 1 BOOK ($5.00 + $2.50)
For order shipped outside the US, add $5.00 per item

___ X ADD $5.00 S. & H. OR EACH ITEM ON ORDER (INTERNATIONAL ORDERS ONLY) $ 5.00 $ ___

Allow up to 21 days for delivery (we will call you about back orders if any)

TOTAL: $ ___

Fax a copy of this order to: 1-888-317-6767 or Int'l + 416-352-5126
or mail to: Rhino Publishing, S.A. Attention: PTY 5048 P.O. Box 025724, Miami, FL., 33102 USA
Digital E-books also available online: www.rhinopublish.com

Printed in the United States
74278LV00003BC/114

9 789962 636106